Preventing Cancer the Natural Way

By Chris Canberra

publication of the trademark is without permission or backing by the trademark owner. All trademarks and brands within this book are for clarifying purposes only and are the owned by the owners themselves, not affiliated with this document.

Acknowledgement

I want to thank you and congratulate you for downloading the book, *"Preventing Cancer The Natural Way"*.

This book contains useful information that will help you be more conscious of your living and how to prevent cancer from a natural approach.

Thanks again for downloading this book, I hope you enjoy it!

Cancer: Beginner's Guide to Preventing Cancer the Natural Way

Introduction

The cancer industry is easily the most lucrative industry in the world today. Thousands of businesses are successfully making a profit from the current $125 billion in medical costs for cancer patients alone. However, various research conducted around the world prove that there are alternative ways of preventing cancer using natural means. Yet the cancer industry, which employs millions and earns even more, continues to prosper while trying to hide the fact that cancer can be prevented.

Simply put, the cancer industry is earning too much money to allow a cure to be found. But natural cures and preventive measures are all around us; all one needs to do is to know where to look.

In this book, we will explore cancer – discuss what it's about, who's at risk, and how you can prevent it without spending millions of dollars.

I.   Introduction to Cancer

Cancer is the collective term given to a broad range of diseases where the body's cells divide uncontrollably. Normal cells can divide in an orderly method: when these cells are damaged or old, new cells grow to take their place. On the other hand, cancer cells tend to crowd normal cells, making it difficult for the body to function the way it should. When cells become abnormal, the damaged or old cells that should have died survive, while new cells grow even if they are not needed. When these extra cells continue to divide, they may form a growth called a tumor. Many kinds of cancers result in a solid tumor or a mass of tissue, although others, such as leukemia or cancer of the blood, do not.

The human body contains trillions of cells, and cancer can begin anywhere: lungs, colon, blood, or even the bone. Many cancers are similar to each other although they differ in how their cells grow, and how they spread around the body.

There are two kinds of tumors: malignant and benign. Malignant refers to tumors that are cancerous and thus can invade surrounding tissues. When tumors grow, some cancer cells can travel around the body through the lymph system or blood, and form a new tumor elsewhere. Benign tumors do not spread into nearby tissues, although they can sometimes grow into large sizes. Benign tumors may be removed through surgery and oftentimes do not grow back although in some instances malignant tumors do. Most benign tumors are not fatal unless it is located in the brain.

Symptoms of Cancer

Because cancer refers to a wide range of diseases, the signs and symptoms vary greatly depending on the location of the cancer, its size, how much it has affected the tissue or organ, and if it has metastasized (spread). When cancer grows, it can cause added pressure or pain to nearby nerves, organs, or blood vessels. If the cancer is a critical location such as the brain, small tumors can already cause symptoms. Some forms of cancer are easier to identify, such as breast or skin cancer, because they form distinguishable lumps outside or underneath the skin.

Some cancers don't show signs or symptoms until they are already quite large. Certain cancers may result in weight loss, fatigue, or fever because the excess cells use the body's energy reserves or release substances that affect how the body converts energy from food. Cancer may also cause the immune system to produce these symptoms.

The general signs of cancer may be difficult to detect because more often than not they do not mean that one has cancer. However, if these symptoms are persistent and do not go away, it's best to see a doctor:

- Fever
- Fatigue
- Unexplained weight loss

- Changes in skin color
- Pain

Treatment

Cancer treatment is always more effective in cases where it is identified early especially when it is smaller and hasn't yet metastasized.

Doctors can perform surgery to remove the cancer as well as other body parts that are affected by the cancer. It is common to remove part or the entire breast in cases of breast cancer. Prostate glands may be removed for prostate cancer.

Chemotherapy utilizes drugs to kill cancer cells and preventing them from dividing. Chemotherapy drugs are powerful and can affect many other growing and healthy cells. This may result in side effects such as fatigue, muscle pain, headaches, stomach pain, pain caused by nerve damage, oral sores, nausea, diarrhea, vomiting, changes in cognitive ability, fertility issues, blood disorders, hair loss, and appetite loss to name a few.

Radiation therapy uses high-energy x-rays to destroy and slow down the growth of cancer cells. It may be used either alone or in conjunction with chemotherapy or surgery. Radiation may result in side effects such as fatigue, skin problems, and the possibility of developing cancer again later on. In addition, the side effects borne from radiation tend to be localized depending on the area that radiation therapy is targeting.

Prognosis

The prognosis for cancer depends on several factors:

- Type of cancer
- Location of cancer in the body
- Stage of cancer
- If the cancer has spread
- Patient's age and status of health prior to cancer

- How the patient responds to treatment
- The cancer's grade

II.   Risk Factors

It can be difficult to explain why one person gets cancer and another doesn't. However, research shows that risk factors can increase the chances that a person may develop cancer at some point in their life. Cancer risk factors include behaviors as well as exposure to substances or chemicals, which are controllable. However, certain cancer risk factors, such as family history and age, cannot be controlled.

In this chapter, we will explore the most widely studied suspected risk factors for cancer. Avoiding exposure to controllable risk factors can lower your risk of developing some cancers.

1. **Age**: The average age for cancer diagnosis is 66 years old; thus older age increases one's proclivity to developing cancer although it can occur at any age. Certain kinds of cancers such as neuroblastoma are more prevalent in children rather than adults.
2. **Alcohol use**: Alcohol consumption can increase risk for throat, mouth, liver, larynx, and breast cancer. When alcohol is combined with tobacco use, cancer risk skyrockets. However with certain cancer-fighting properties such as resveratrol present in red wine, recommended consumption is up to 2 glasses daily.
3. **Hormones**: Although hormones play an important role in men and women, estrogen has been associated with an increase in cancer risk. Women who take combined menopausal hormone therapy which contains estrogen plus progestin can increase the risk of breast cancer. Research shows that breast cancer risk is linked to the progesterone and estrogen produced by the ovaries. Prolonged exposure to these hormones, such as when a

woman starts menstruation at an early age, never giving birth, going through a late menopause, or when the first pregnancy is at a later age, all increases a woman's risk of acquiring breast cancer.

4. **Obesity**: Overweight people are at risk for several cancers while staying at a healthy weight and maintaining an active lifestyle reduces the risk of cancer.

5. **Radiation**: Exposure to ionizing radiation found in x-rays, radon, gamma rays and other sources of high energy radiation can damage DNA and result in cancer. Non-ionizing forms of radiation such as those found in cell phones as well as magnetic fields are not intense enough to cause DNA damage or cancer.

    a. Radon is a form of radioactive gas found in soil and rocks. People living in areas that contain high levels of radon in its soil and rocks are more vulnerable to developing lung cancer later on.

    b. High energy radiation sources include medical procedures that utilize x-rays, positron emission tomography (PET) scan, and computed tomography (CT) scans; alpha particles, beta particles, gamma rays, and neutrons are strong enough to result in DNA damage as well as cancer. Aside from hospital procedures, high energy radiation can also be released as a result of accidents in nuclear power plants.

6. **Sunlight**: Exposure to the sun and tanning booths gives off ultraviolet (UV) rays which can cause skin damage and skin cancer. The amount of time spent under the sun and in tanning beds should be limited by people of all ages to reduce risk of developing skin cancer. In addition, UV radiation can also be reflected by water, ice, sand, and snow; thus, anyone exposed should use proper protection by means of protective clothing and sunscreen with at least a sun protection factor of 15. Other useful ways of limiting UV radiation outdoors is by wearing long-sleeved clothing, sunglasses, and wide-brimmed hats.

7. **Tobacco**: Tobacco use and cigarette smoking is the number one cause of cancer worldwide. People who are often around others who smoke cigarettes are also at risk of developing cancer due to exposure to second-hand smoke because the smoke emitted by cigarettes contains enough chemicals to cause damage to DNA. Tobacco use can result in several cancers including larynx, lung, esophagus, mouth, bladder, liver, kidney and many more. Those who use smokeless tobacco are also at risk of developing cancers of the mouth, pancreas, and throat. When it comes to tobacco use, zero tolerance is recommended for anyone who wants to reduce their cancer risk because there is no such thing as a safe amount of tobacco to smoke.

III.   Preventing Cancer Through Natural Means

Despite what the cancer industry says, it is possible to prevent cancer naturally. The key to preventing cancer is in your lifestyle: the food you eat, the amount of exercise you get, the chemicals and toxins your body is exposed to, and your sleeping habits all play a role. The good news is that all of these factors can be controlled. It is also important to remember that while there is no one food that will prevent cancer altogether, successful prevention lies in the combination of efforts that are described here later on.

Cancer doesn't develop overnight but by making these changes to your lifestyle, you can significantly reduce your risk of developing it later on.

a.   Diet and Nutrition

Food contains a variety of components that aid in cancer prevention: these include vitamins, minerals, macronutrients, and phytonutrients from plants. The National Cancer Institute states that as much as 80% of cancers are due to specific lifestyle factors; 30% of these are due to smoking and as much as 50% are associated with a poor diet. What you eat and what you don't eat can have a significant effect on your overall health. Certain foods can increase your risk of cancer; similarly, you may be neglecting important foods that can dramatically reduce your risk.

In addition, research has also been conducted that emphasizes there is a link between an acidic body and cancer risk. Cancer, as well as many other preventable diseases such as diabetes and arthritis, can only grow in an acidic environment and also cannot survive in an alkaline environment. Those who develop cancer have acidic bodies and low pH levels. Certain foods can either increase the acidity in one's body and thus an ideal diet for cancer prevention is one that raises the body's alkalinity.

What To Avoid

- Genetically modified organisms (GMO's) and pesticides: GMO's may be plants or animals whose DNA has been manipulated to be resistant to pesticides. Studies have shown that farmers who are exposed to genetically modified crops and pesticides have a higher incidence of developing cancer. Consumption of genetically modified animals or crops can also increase one's risk of developing certain cancers such as brain tumors, breast cancer, and leukemia among others.
- Processed meat: Processed meat refers to any meat that has been altered to change its taste or extend its shelf life. The most common methods used in processed meat include curing, smoking, or adding preservatives. Popular forms of processed meat include corned beef, hotdogs, sausages, bacon, ham, canned meat, beef jerky, and meat-based sauces. Not only is meat an acid-forming food, but the chemicals used in processing these meats are highly carcinogenic. Cooking in high temperatures such as barbecue or grilling also creates carcinogenic chemicals. While no red meat is best, medium or

rare is a better choice. Any food that is charred, even toast, should be avoided.

- Farmed fish: Dioxins, toxaphene, PCB's, and dieldrin- all cancer-causing substances have been found in high concentrations in farmed salmon which is present on most grocery store shelves and served in restaurants. Other varieties of farm-bred fish, including tilapia, contain high amounts of pesticides and antibiotics that are used to keep them alive.

- Refined sugar: Commonly known as sucrose, refined sugar is derived from sugar beet or sugar cane. Sucrose is present in white and brown sugar that is used to make cakes, cookies, and to sweeten coffee. Refined sugar is also found in high-fructose corn syrup which is present in flavored yogurt, salad dressings, and tomato sauce. These sugars are linked to obesity-related cancers and its consumption also increases the body's acidity levels.

- Canned food: Cans contain a carcinogen bisphenol-A (BPA) which has been linked to breast and prostate cancer incidence. It is a synthetic estrogen that can disrupt hormones even with minimal exposure. Canned tomatoes contain the highest levels of BPA because its high acidity causes BPA to leech from the cans. BPA is also present in a number of household products including utensils, microwave ovenware, and some baby bottles.

- Aspartame: Commonly found in artificial sweeteners such as NutraSweet and Equal, aspartame has been linked to several illnesses as well as cancer. Research has shown that the chemicals contained in aspartame and other artificial sweeteners produce a deadly toxin in the body called DKP which in turn can produce carcinogens when it is being processed in the body.

- "Diet" and "Low-fat" food: Any frozen or pre-packaged food that is labeled "diet" or "low-fat" either contain aspartame, refined ingredients, high levels of sodium, and artificial flavoring to give it taste.

- <u>Excess salt:</u> While salt consumption is necessary for health, too much salt can result in cancer and many other illnesses. The recommended dosage for salt should be less than 1,500 milligrams of sodium per day.
- <u>Junk food:</u> The consumption of junk food puts you at risk for cancer, obesity, and a host of other diseases:
    - Soft drinks and soda: The caramel food coloring that is widely used to give the beverage its brownish hue produces 4-MEI, which is a carcinogen. In addition, soft drinks contain high amounts of sugar in various forms; the consumption of sugar alters the body's pH in the intestines and increase acidity.
    - Snacks that contain trans-fat: The most common snacks containing trans-fat include French fries, potato chips, deep fried foods, margarine, frosting, shortening, microwave popcorn, chips (tortilla, potato, corn), and creamer.

What to Eat

- <u>Fruits and vegetables:</u> Consuming fresh produce in all colors is an ideal way to ensure that you are getting maximum protection from cancer. Fruits and vegetables are rich in antioxidants including vitamins C and E, beta-carotene, and selenium which protect the body from cancer and aid in efficient functioning of organs and tissues.

As a general rule of thumb, fruits and vegetables have more potent cancer-fighting properties when they are altered as little as possible from the way they came out of the ground. This means that the less they are peeled or cooked, the better. Going organic is a better option especially if you intend to consume the skin of a fruit or vegetable as it is the skin exposed to pesticides. Also, while there is no need to go completely vegetarian in order to prevent cancer, you can achieve a balance by ensuring you add whole fruits and vegetables to each meal.

- Whole grains: Whole grains are important sources of fiber, protein, and magnesium. There are several kinds of whole grains to choose from, all of which are hearty, filling and flavorful. These include whole-wheat bread, corn, brown rice, barley, oatmeal, faro, millet, and others. Whole grains are more nutritious because they contain cancer-fighting phytochemicals while helping keep the digestive system functioning optimally. Other healthy compounds that are found in whole grains include saponins, lignans, flavonoids, phytic acid, and protease inhibitors.

- Legumes: Split peas, dry beans, and lentils are not only an excellent source of fiber and protein, but they are also rich in cancer-fighting compounds that include: lignans, saponins, resistant starch, and several phytochemicals.

- Coffee: A cup of good quality coffee may be an important source of antioxidant phytochemicals and riboflavin. However, the amount of antioxidants in coffee depends largely on how the coffee is prepared as well as how the beans are grown.

b. Top Foods with Cancer-Fighting Properties

Adding these foods to your daily diet will help boost immunity and provide you with nutrients and vitamins all while reducing your risk of cancer.

1. **Berries** are rich in potent antioxidants that fight cell-damaging free radicals. Berries also contain natural components that prevent cancer from spreading or growing.
2. **Tomatoes** are rich in lycopene, an antioxidant that may reduce the risk for certain cancers including breast and prostate.
3. **Green tea** contains catechins which are associated with a lower risk of cancer. Sipping a cup or two of green tea a day also prevents free radicals from causing cell damage.
4. **Turmeric** is an orange colored spice which is widely used in Indian cuisine. It contains curcumin which helps inhibit the growth of cancer cells and protects the liver from cirrhosis. Turmeric may be taken in capsule form or added as a powder into curries and other dishes.

5. **Grapes** contain an antioxidant known as resveratrol which may be beneficial in inhibiting cancer growth. Resveratrol is found in grape juice as well as red wine and has been shown to lower risk of prostate cancer.

6. **Dark chocolate** that contains at least 70% cocoa or cacao is rich in therapeutic polyphenols and antioxidants that help fight cancer. Catechins, in particular, are also present in dark chocolates.

7. **Nuts and seeds** can help reduce risk of developing certain cancers, particularly those found in the list below:

   Healthiest nuts:
   Walnuts
   Almonds
   Pecans
   Brazil nuts
   Cedar nuts

   Healthiest seeds:
   Hemp
   Sunflower
   Sesame
   Pumpkin
   Chia

c. Top Alkaline Foods

These foods can be integrated into your daily diet to help your body attain an alkaline state:

1. Cruciferous vegetables are easy to prepare in nutritious recipes while others can be tossed into a blender to supercharge your smoothie. These include:

- Arugula
- Basil
- Beet greens
- Bokchoy
- Broccoli
- Brussel sprouts
- Cabbage
- Celery
- Chard
- Spinach
- Kale

2. Root vegetables can be eaten raw, steamed, roasted, or sautéed. These include:

- Beets
- Carrots
- Garlic
- Ginger
- Kohlrabi
- Onion
- Parsnips
- Sweet potato
- Turnips
- Yuca root

3. Leafy greens are not only alkaline vegetables but are also packed with vitamins and nutrients. Their alkalizing qualities are

more beneficial when eaten raw but light consuming them lightly steamed or marinated will also do. An effective and delicious way of consuming leafy greens is also by adding them to juices or smoothies.

- Cabbage
- Collard greens
- Dandelion greens
- Kale
- Mustard greens
- Romaine lettuce
- Turnip greens
- Spinach
- Swiss chard
- Watercress

4. **Lemons** are recognized as a highly alkaline food which is also extremely versatile. Drinking lemon water daily is an easy way to maximize the alkalizing effects of lemon on the body. Lemon juice can be used to season many dishes and salads.

5. **Cucumbers** make a great base for soups and can easily be added to juices and smoothies. They are one of the most alkaline vegetables and are also rich in vitamins A and C, manganese, potassium, magnesium, and folate. Cucumbers are water-rich and make filling snacks for any time of the day. Cucumber and lemon slices in water will also give you a delicious-tasting alkaline water.

d. Supplements and Super foods

These super foods and vitamins are a great addition to your diet. They are extremely nutritious and possess powerful cancer-fighting properties. Before taking any of these supplements or super foods, it is best to talk to your doctor first.

- **Spirulina**, a blue-green algae, thrives in alkaline warm-water lakes. Spirulina derives its color from the protein phycocyanin, which can slow down the growth of cancer cells. Just like other plants and algae, spirulina is also rich in chlorophyll which has the ability to bind with cancer cells and promote its excretion from the body before they group into colonies and form tumors within the body. Spirulina may be taken in capsule or powder form.

- **Cacao** nibs contain high amounts of flavonoids which may prevent cancer and other illnesses including Alzheimer's. Flavonoids help prevent cellular damage caused by free radicals. In addition, cacao nibs are also rich in fiber, another key nutrient that helps in cancer prevention. Cacao nibs are best enjoyed raw, added to shakes, yogurts, and breakfast bowls.

- **Moringa**, a plant that grows in tropical areas of the world, is highly prized for its medicinal properties. Moringa is a powerful source of vitamin c, vitamin a, iron, calcium, potassium, and protein. In India, moringa plant is cultivated for its anti-tumor, anti-inflammatory, and anti-cancer properties. The plant contains a total of 36 anti-inflammatory agents, making it one of the most potent anti-cancer plants in the world. Moringa may be consumed in capsule, tablet, or powder form.

- **Chlorella** is freshwater seaweed or green algae that are recognized for its cancer-fighting properties. It is an excellent source of chlorophyll, protein, B vitamins, carbohydrates, amino acids, vitamin c, and vitamin e. Chlorella's nutritional content makes it a powerful defense in keeping the immune system strong enough to stave off inflammation and cancer. It is also taken by cancer patients to help their bodies tolerate chemotherapy more effectively. Chlorella is widely used in Japan where its healing qualities are well-known. Chlorella may be taken in capsule, tablet, or powder form.

- **Virgin coconut oil** derived from coconut trees is rich in immune-boosting and cancer-fighting properties. Its potent antioxidant properties have the ability to reverse cellular damage that may result in cancer while providing protection from free radicals. Virgin coconut oil is also rich in lauric acid which helps to kill viruses, bacteria, yeast, and parasites. It is also one of the most versatile oils in the world, providing people with health benefits regardless of which way it is used. Coconut oil is widely used as a cooking oil; it can be heated several times over without producing free radicals thus cooking with coconut oil can reduce cancer risk. Raw, virgin, organic coconut oil is ideal for cancer prevention; it is best taken in raw form orally. It can also be taken in capsule form or added directly to food.

Supplements

- **Coenzyme Q10** may reduce cancer risk while large amounts can inhibit breast cancer growth while boosting immunity. Recommended dosage of CoQ10 for cancer prevention is 100mg per day.
- **Lycopene** supplements help prevent cellular damage caused by free radicals. Research has also shown that taking lycopene supplements may be able to reduce prostate tumors and inhibit growth. Recommended dosage for prostate cancer prevention is 10mg daily even if your diet already contains lycopene-rich foods.

- **Selenium** contains an antioxidant enzyme that helps the liver detoxify cancer-causing toxins. Studies show that 200 micrograms of selenium taken daily can significantly reduce one's risk of developing lung, colon, and prostate cancers.
- **Vitamin K** can reduce the risk for cancers of the liver and the breast. The recommended dosage is 300 micrograms of vitamin K-1 or K-2.

e. Exercise

Regular exercise can significantly reduce the risk of getting several cancers, including breast, bowel, prostate, and womb. Ideally, 30 minutes of rigorous exercise or an hour of moderate activity is recommended.

Physical activity can combat cancer by fighting inflammation and reducing obesity. Inflammation is the immune system's response to injury which is often caused by pathogens. Common characteristics of inflammation include increased blood flow, redness, swelling, and pain. These can occur in wounds outside the body as well as in organs and tissues that are not immediately visible to the human eye. Chronic inflammation can happen even if there is no injury because it results in DNA damage. Studies have shown that humans who experience inflammation for long periods of time are at higher risk of developing cancer. For example, those who suffer from chronic inflammatory bowel diseases such as Crohn's disease are at higher risk for colon cancer. A physically active body produces more antioxidants which are necessary for fighting the free radicals that cause inflammation.

Exercise is also an effective way to deal with stress, which triggers inflammation. Chronic stress can alter immune cells even before they enter the bloodstream, making them ready to fight infection even when there is no injury which then leads to inflammation.

Furthermore, regular exercise is crucial for keeping excess weight off. Obesity is linked to several cancers including breast, esophagus, pancreas, colon, gallbladder, kidney, and endometrium. There are several facts that link obesity with cancer:

- The blood of obese people have been shown to contain higher levels of insulin growth factor 1 (IGF-1) and insulin which has been shown to increase risk for certain cancers.
- Adipose tissue produces excess estrogen, an occurrence that has been tied to endometrial, breast, and other kinds of cancers.
- Obesity leads to chronic sub-level inflammation, which thus increases one's cancer risk.

f. Sleep

Adequate sleep is crucial for disease prevention and ensuring your body is performing at its optimal best. Prolonged periods of impaired sleep have been linked to cancer and quicker growth of tumors. Studies show that men who have difficulties sleeping well had higher incidence of prostate cancer, and inadequate sleep may result in the recurrence of breast cancer while increasing the risk of developing more aggressive forms of breast cancer in women.

Less than 6 hours of sleep a night can increase the risk for colorectal adenoma which can result in cancer. In general, people who sleep less than 6 hours at night increased cancer risk by as much as 50% when compared to those who got at least 7 hours of sleep a night.

Insulin resistance combined with disrupted melatonin production is two primary processes which can increase cancer risk as a result of poor sleep. Furthermore, insufficient sleep decreases the levels of leptin in the body which are necessary for regulating fat resulting in increased levels of ghrelin, a hunger hormone. Therefore, those who don't get adequate sleep are more prone to overeating and gaining excess weight. Overweight women are most affected by the insulin resistance and weight gain risk factors. Breast cancer is the most prevalent form of cancer in women, yet women who are obese are as much as 60% more prone due to the insulin resistance that occurs as a result of poor sleep habits. Breast cancers are fueled by the body's estrogen production which increases when a woman has more fat.

In addition, those who work the night shift are at higher risk of developing cancer and a host of other illnesses. Hormone disruptions are likely the primary cause of cancer in those who work night shifts. Even if you live a healthy lifestyle and eat the right foods, getting inadequate sleep can discount all of these and still put you at risk for cancer.

g.   Environmental toxins

1.   Household cleaners

People oftentimes don't realize how many chemicals they are allowing themselves to be exposed to simply by using household cleaners. Switching to natural and environmentally safe household products is an easy and inexpensive way to make your home cancer-free. It's also relatively easy and inexpensive to make your own natural household cleaners using lemons, vodka, soap, or vinegar mixed diluted in water.

Several of the chemicals found in common household cleaners can cause cancer and thus any product containing these should be avoided:

- Synthetic musks
- Terpenes
- Phenol
- Phthalates
- Benzene

- Petroleum solvents
- Butyl cellosolve
- Nonylphenol ethoxylates (NPE)
- Styrene
- 1,4-diclorobenzene
- Formaldehyde
- Triclosan

2. Beauty Products

Personal care products may seem beneficial to use at first, but once you start examining product labels you may be surprised to find cancer-causing chemicals lurking in your shampoo or body lotion. Skin exposure to these chemicals increases is even worse than ingesting them because the skin absorbs them immediately and it goes directly into the bloodstream.

The most common chemicals found in personal and beauty care products to avoid include:

- Sodium lauryl sulfate (SLS)
- Paraben
- Musks
- 1,4 –Dioxane
- Phthalates
- Antibacterials
- Mineral oil
- Paraffin
- Petroleum
- Hydroquinone
- Mercury
- Lead
- Formaldehyde

• Nano particles

A good rule of thumb when it comes to personal care products is if you wouldn't eat it then it probably isn't safe enough to use on your skin. Use organic, all-natural, and vegan products on your face and body whenever possible.

IV.   Conclusion

Cancer is a disease dreaded by people worldwide, understandably so as it causes millions of deaths every year. The cancer industry adds to the stigma, given the fact that the business is considered lucrative. Too little is done to educate people on how cancer can be prevented naturally and thus many people end up feeling helpless when it comes to understanding what changes can be made in order to reduce one's risk for cancer. Keep in mind that more than half of all cancer deaths could have easily been prevented by taking simple steps such as quitting cigarettes, eating the proper food, getting enough exercise, and living a healthy lifestyle. These things are not rocket-science – but by taking the first step forward in understanding what you can change today, you are well on your way to a cancer-free life.

Thank you again for downloading this book!

If you enjoyed this book, would you mind kindly providing us with a review on Amazon?

Because we're happy that you bought our book, we would like to offer you a special gift for a free book.

Simply go to the following link:

http://healthylivingoffer.weebly.com